DETOXIFICATION DIET PLAN GUIDE BOOK

The Ultimate Detox Diet: Foods Restoring and Purifying Your Body

REX LEWIS

Table of Contents

Introduction

Detoxification, sometimes called detox, is the method by which the body gets rid of or balances out harmful substances. These substances may consist of medications, metabolic byproducts, toxins from the environment, and other hazardous substances. Although the liver is the primary organ involved in detoxification, the kidneys, skin, lungs, and gastrointestinal system are also important in the removal of toxins.

The Following Are Crucial Ideas In Detoxifying Understanding:

1. Liver Purpose:

• An essential organ for detoxification is the liver. It breaks down and changes toxins into substances that the body can quickly eliminate that are soluble in water.

• The liver goes through two primary stages of detoxification: Phase I and Phase II. Phase I involves the breakdown of toxins into intermediate forms; Phase II involves additional processing of these intermediates to make them water-soluble and excretable.

2. Kidney Function:

• Waste materials and poisons are filtered out of the bloodstream by the kidneys, which results in urine. Maintaining adequate hydration is essential for renal function and effective removal of toxins.

3. The Digestive System

• The process of detoxification involves the gastrointestinal tract's removal of waste materials. Dietary fiber aids in the binding of toxins and makes it easier for the feces to remove them.

4. Lungs and Skin:

• Toxins are eliminated by sweating the skin and breathing them out of the lungs. Exercise and saunas are two activities that can increase sweating and improve the removal of some pollutants.

5. Programs and Diets for Detoxification:

• It's common to hear about diets and programs that help the body's natural detoxification processes. These could include following a certain diet plan, fasting, or consuming particular foods or supplements that are thought to help with detoxification.

6. Hydration and Water:

• Water improves kidney function and aids in the flushing out of waste materials through urine, making it crucial for the removal of toxins.

7. Natural Detoxifying Ingredients:

• It's thought that some drugs and meals aid in the detoxification process. For instance, certain herbs may strengthen the liver, while antioxidants in fruits and vegetables may aid in the neutralization of free radicals.

8. Use Detox Programs with Care:

• Although certain detoxification techniques can be helpful, lengthy or intense detoxification regimens carry some risk and should be used with caution. It's crucial to speak with medical experts before beginning any kind of extensive detoxification program.

9. Personal Differences:

• Individual differences in exposure to pollutants, general health, and heredity can all affect how beneficial and necessary detoxification is.

It's important to remember that detoxification is a normal function of the human body. Maintaining a healthy lifestyle with a balanced diet, frequent exercise, and adequate water can help the body's natural detoxification processes. Seeking individualised assistance from a healthcare professional is recommended for those with particular health issues or problems.

CHAPTER ONE
Describe Detoxification.

The Physiological Or Medical Process Of Removing Hazardous Substances From The Human Body Is Called Detoxification. The Phrase Is Frequently Used To Refer To The Body's Innate Capacity To Neutralize Or Get Rid Of Dangerous Chemicals, Such As Medications, Waste Products From Metabolism, And Contaminants From The Environment. The Liver, Kidneys, Skin, Lungs, And Gastrointestinal Tract Are The Main Organs That Are Involved In Detoxification.

This Is A Condensed Explanation Of Detoxification:

1. Liver Impoverishment:

• An essential organ for detoxification is the liver. Toxins are broken down and changed into forms the body can quickly expel. Phase I and Phase II are the two primary stages of this process.

2. Kidney Function:

• To create urine, the kidneys filter the blood, eliminating waste materials and extra fluid. This procedure aids in the body's removal of poisons that are soluble in water.

3. The Digestive System

• Through the digestion and elimination of waste items, the gastrointestinal system contributes to detoxification. Dietary fiber helps bind toxins and make it easier for the body to eliminate them through bowel movements.

4. Lungs and Skin:

• Toxins are eliminated by sweating the skin and breathing them out of the lungs. For example, exercising and using saunas can improve one's ability to sweat.

5. Organic Detoxification:

• The body has natural detoxification processes that are assisted by a variety of nutrients and chemicals from a balanced diet. The body has built-in mechanisms to cope with toxins. For example, antioxidants aid in the neutralization of free radicals.

6. Drinking Plenty of Water

• Sustaining detoxification requires adequate fluids. Water promotes the general health of the detoxifying organs and aids in the elimination of pollutants through urine.

Although the body naturally detoxifies, the word "detox" is also frequently associated with diets, cleanses, or programs that promote detoxification. These could entail fasting, certain dietary adjustments, or the use of substances that are meant to help the body detoxify. It's crucial to remember that there is frequently no scientific proof for the effectiveness of many commercial detox products and programs.

Seeking advice from medical professionals is advised prior to starting any kind of detox treatment. Extensive or intense detoxification procedures might not be necessary for everyone and include dangers. Sustainable lifestyle decisions, such as eating a well-balanced diet, drinking plenty of water, and exercising frequently, can improve general health and assist the body's inherent detoxification processes.

Detox Diet Benefits

Detox diets are frequently advertised as a means of removing toxins from the body, enhancing general health, and increasing vitality. It's vital to remember that scientific research on the precise benefits of detox diets is scarce and frequently inconclusive, despite some anecdotal evidence and personal testimonies to the contrary. Some possible advantages of detox diets that supporters have mentioned are as follows:

1. Enhanced Vitality:

• Proponents of detox diets assert that people may feel more energised and vital by cutting out processed meals, sweets, and coffee and concentrating on foods high in nutrients.

2. Loss of Weight:

• A detox diet may cause some people to lose weight; this is mostly because they are consuming less calories and losing water weight. It's possible that this weight loss won't last in the long run, though.

3. Enhanced Digestive Health:

• Whole, plant-based meals that are high in fiber and support improved digestive health are frequently the focus of detox diets. A higher fiber diet can promote regular bowel movements and aid in the body's waste removal.

4. Decreased Inflammation:

• Anti-inflammatory foods, like fruits and vegetables, are emphasized in some detox diets, as they may help lower inflammation in the body.

5. Improved Mental Acuity and Concentration:

• After going on detox diets, some people claim to have more attention and mental clarity. This could be related to things like drinking enough of water, eating foods high in nutrients, and cutting back on things like coffee.

6. Skin Enhancement:

• Some people may see cleaner skin after following a detox diet. This might result from drinking more water, eating fewer processed meals, and maybe getting rid of some allergies.

7. Promotes Optimal Eating Practices:

• Consuming natural, unprocessed foods is frequently encouraged whereas consuming processed and sugary foods is discouraged in detox diets. The focus on nutritious eating practices may have long-term advantages for general health.

It's crucial to proceed cautiously when considering these potential advantages and keep the following things in mind:

• **Lack of Scientific Consensus:** There is little scientific proof of the particular advantages of detox diets, and further study is required to determine their effectiveness and long-term effects.

- **Individual Variability:** Everyone reacts differently to detox diets. While some people could see favorable changes, others might not notice any changes at all or might even have unpleasant side effects.

- **Possible Risks:** Prolonged or intense detox diets increase the risk of muscle loss, vitamin shortages, and other health problems. It's important to speak with a medical expert before making any significant dietary adjustments.

In conclusion, while some people may benefit temporarily from detox diets, it is still unclear what will happen to their general health in the long run. In general, it is advised to promote health and well-being by eating in a balanced and sustainable manner, drinking plenty of water, and getting regular exercise. Before making any major dietary or lifestyle changes, always get medical advice.

CHAPTER TWO
Getting Ready for Your Detox

It's crucial to approach any detox you're thinking about with serious thought and preparation. Remember that different people will interpret the term "detox" differently; it can refer to anything from brief dietary changes to more intensive cleansing regimens. To help you get ready for a detox, consider the following general advice:

1. Speak with a Medical Professional:

• See a healthcare provider prior to beginning any detox program, particularly if you are taking medication or have pre-existing medical issues. Personalized recommendations depending on your health situation can be given by them.

2. Establish Your Objectives:

•   Clearly state your intentions regarding the detox. Having clear goals will help you select the right detox plan and track your success, whether your goal is weight loss, more energy, or overall well-being.

3. Select a Reasonable and Safe Detox Plan:

• Steer clear of severe or unduly stringent detoxification regimens since these may result in dietary deficits or other health problems. Choose realistic, well-balanced diets that feature a range of nutrient-dense foods.

4. Drinking Plenty of Water

• It's important to drink enough of water whilst on a detox. Water aids in the body's natural elimination of toxins and assists its detoxification processes. Additionally, think about adding herbal infusions and teas.

5. Organize Your Meals:

• Schedule your meals in advance if your detox calls for any dietary adjustments. To supply vital nutrients, make sure they are well-balanced and include a range of fruits, vegetables, whole grains, and lean proteins.

6. Gradual Changeover:

• Consider transitioning gradually rather than making abrupt, severe changes to your diet if your detox calls for considerable food adjustments. This may lessen the chance of experiencing withdrawal symptoms or stomach problems.

7. Take Out Sugar and Processed Foods:

• Eliminating processed foods, sweets, and caffeine is a common step in detoxification programs. To facilitate the transition, begin cutting back on these substances a few days before beginning the detox.

8. Fill Up on Foods High in Nutrients:

• Make sure you keep a range of nutrient-dense foods on hand, including fresh produce, lean meats, nuts, and seeds. Maintaining your detox plan will be simpler if you have these solutions on hand.

9. Consciously Consuming Food:

• When on detox, eat with awareness. Take note of your body's signals of hunger and fullness, and enjoy every bite. This may encourage a more positive connection with eating.

10. Encouragement Setting:

• Tell your loved ones about your detoxification strategy and ask for their help. A welcoming atmosphere can help to simplify the procedure.

11. Pay Attention to Your Body:

• During the detox, observe how your body reacts. See a medical expert if you suffer from unpleasant symptoms or discomfort.

12. After-Detox Phase:

• After the detox, schedule a gradual return to your regular diet. Reintroducing some meals suddenly can cause stomach problems.

Recall that everyone's body has natural detoxification processes, so drastic measures may not always be required. Three essential elements of a healthy lifestyle are normal physical activity, a well-balanced diet centered on whole foods, and adequate water. Prioritize your health and wellbeing at all times, and seek medical advice before making big dietary or lifestyle changes.

Different Detox Diets

There are many different types of detox diets, but they all generally entail altering one's food to remove toxins from the body. It's crucial to remember that there is no scientific proof for the effectiveness and safety of various detox diets, and that each person will react differently. These are a few popular categories of detox diets:

1. Juice Fasting:

• During a juice cleanse, participants only drink fresh fruit and vegetable juices for a predetermined amount of time. The goal is to replenish the body with vitamins, minerals, and antioxidants while providing some much-needed rest for the digestive system.

2. Water Fasting:

• Water fasting entails giving up all meals and consuming just water for a predetermined amount of time. It seeks to facilitate cleansing and give the digestive system a break. Long-term water fasting ought to be carried out under medical guidance.

3. Whole Foods Fasting:

• The goal of this strategy is to cut out processed foods, added sugars, and possible allergies from the diet. Rather, they eat entire, high-nutrient foods including fruits, vegetables, lean meats, and whole grains.

4. Raw Food Fasting:

• Consuming solely uncooked, raw foods—such as fruits, vegetables, nuts, and seeds—is known as a raw food detox. Proponents contend that eating a raw food diet promotes detoxification and that heating destroys minerals and enzymes.

5. Diets Based On Elimination:

• These diets call for the temporary elimination of particular food groups that are assumed to be the source of allergies or sensitivities. Dairy, processed sugars, gluten, and soy are common foods to avoid.

6. The Lemonade Diet, or Master Cleanse:

• The Master Cleanse calls for consuming a mixture of water, lemon juice, maple syrup, and cayenne pepper for a predetermined amount of time. It is frequently applied for brief detoxification.

7. Periodic Fasting:

• Intermittent fasting is a type of eating and fasting that alternates, albeit it's not strictly a detox diet. Intermittent fasting has some supporters who claim it can help with detoxification and general wellness.

8. Alkaline Diet:

• Eating foods that alkalize the body, like fruits, vegetables, and some nuts, is the focus of the alkaline diet. Advocates assert that detoxification is supported by an alkaline atmosphere.

9. Tea Detox, also known as Teatox:

• Teatox is the practice of consuming herbal teas that are said to have cleansing qualities. These teas frequently include liver-supporting herbs like milk thistle, ginger, and dandelion.

10. Colon Cleanses:

• To eliminate waste and toxins from the colon, colon cleanses may use techniques like colonic irrigation or the use of herbal supplements. In the medical world, there is disagreement over colon cleanses' effectiveness and safety.

11. Supplements for Detoxification:

• To aid the body's detoxification processes, several detox diets call for the usage of supplements like herbal extracts or detox tablets. The efficacy of these supplements varies, though.

It's important to use caution when implementing detox diets and to think about speaking with a healthcare provider before making any big dietary adjustments. There are hazards associated with extreme or extended detoxification methods, and not all detox diets have been proven to be effective by science. Promoting health and well-being typically involves adopting sustainable lifestyle choices like eating a balanced diet, drinking plenty of water, and exercising frequently.

CHAPTER THREE
The Plan for Detox Diet

A detox diet plan usually entails altering one's diet to cut out specific foods or food groups that are thought to be involved in the build-up of toxins in the body. Any detox regimen should be followed carefully and ideally with the assistance of a healthcare provider. The fundamental idea of a detox diet plan is provided below, however individual needs and results may differ:

1. Preparing for Detox:

• A few days before to beginning the detox, gradually cut back on processed foods, sweets, caffeine, and alcohol.

• Drink more water to maintain proper hydration.

2. Time Spent on Detox:

• The length of detox diets might vary. While some prefer longer programs, others may pick shorter detox plans (such as those lasting three to seven days). Extended or severe detoxification, however, needs to be handled carefully.

3. Emphasis on Complete, Plant-Based Diets:

• Place a focus on whole grains, legumes, nuts, seeds, and fruits and vegetables. These foods are high in antioxidants, fiber, vitamins, and minerals.

4. Drinking Plenty of Water

• Stay hydrated throughout the day to aid the body's natural cleansing procedures.

• Add herbal teas, such green or dandelion tea, which some people think have cleansing qualities.

5. Get Rid of Possible Allergens:

• In certain detox protocols, common allergies or sensitivities like gluten, dairy, soy, and processed sugars are temporarily eliminated.

6. Sources of Lean Protein:

• Include lean protein foods to enhance muscular health and supply vital amino acids, such as fish, poultry, tofu, or lentils.

7. Eat Less Processed Food:

• Avoid packaged and processed foods because they could have preservatives and additives.

• Choose entire, fresh foods to get the most nutrients possible.

8. Cut Down on Salt Consumption:

• Eat fewer items high in salt to assist prevent water retention.

9. Control of Portion:

• Be mindful of portion sizes to prevent overindulgence and promote intestinal well-being.

10. Probiotics: To promote gut health, eat foods high in probiotics, such as yogurt or fermented vegetables.

11. Exercise: To promote general well-being, partake in regular physical activity like yoga, jogging, or walking.

12. Post-Detox Transition: - Watch how your body reacts by progressively adding the things you gave up back into your diet. - For long-term health, think about implementing a sustainable and balanced dietary plan.

13. Listen to Your Body: - Throughout the detox, observe how your body reacts. If you encounter negative consequences, speak with a medical expert.

It's crucial to remember that while detox diets may help some people in the short term, it's still unclear what the long-term impacts and overall influence will be on health. Plans for detoxing should be carefully considered, as there may be hazards associated with severe or protracted detoxification procedures.

It's best to speak with a healthcare provider before beginning any detox plan to be sure the strategy is safe and appropriate for your particular requirements and objectives. A healthcare professional can provide advice on leading a sustainable lifestyle that promotes general health and wellbeing.

Improving Your Experience with Detox

Numerous practices can be added to your detox regimen, whether you're thinking about doing one or have already begun, to improve your experience and aid your body's natural detoxification processes. Here are some pointers:

1. Maintain Hydration:

• To aid in detoxifying, water is necessary. It facilitates the body's removal of poisons. Drink as much water as possible during the day, and think about flavoring it with slices of cucumber or lemon.

2. Add Foods That Are Detoxifying:

• Include foods like leafy greens, garlic, ginger, turmeric, and cruciferous vegetables (broccoli, cabbage, and kale) that are known for their detoxifying qualities. These meals are rich in antioxidants and promote healthy liver function.

3. Herbal Teas:

• Sip herbal teas, such ginger, green, or dandelion tea, that may have cleansing effects. These teas aid in the removal of pollutants and may have diuretic properties.

4. Encourage The Health Of Your Liver:

• Eat foods that help the liver, such as leafy greens, artichokes, beets, and carrots. Compounds in these foods facilitate the process of detoxification.

5. Incorporate High-Fibre Foods:

• Fiber promotes regular bowel motions, which facilitate waste removal. Consume a diet high in fruits, vegetables, whole grains, and legumes, among other fiber-rich foods.

6. Exercise Frequently:

• Exercise frequently to encourage sweating, lymphatic drainage, and circulation. Exercise can improve the body's natural detoxification mechanisms and promote general well-being.

7. Hot Tubs or Saunas:

• Sweating is another way the body gets rid of toxins, and saunas and hot baths can encourage it. But it's crucial to avoid overheating and to stay hydrated.

8. Techniques for Deep Breathing and Relaxation:

• Reducing stress is essential for general health. To help manage stress, try deep breathing exercises, yoga, or meditation. Prolonged stress might hinder the body's ability to detoxify.

9. Using A Dry Brush:

• Dry brushing the skin before to a shower has the potential to encourage detoxification and activate the lymphatic system. Apply a natural bristle brush on your skin and gently scrub in circular strokes.

10. Restful Sleep:

• Make sure you receive enough restful sleep. The body goes through several detoxification and repair processes while you sleep. Try to get seven to nine hours each night.

11. Consciously Consuming Food:

• Eat mindfully by being aware of your body's signals of hunger and fullness.

To improve digestion, thoroughly chew your meal and enjoy every bite.

12. Think About Probiotics:

• Probiotics have been shown to improve gut health, which is related to general health. Think about consuming more foods high in probiotics, such as fermented veggies, kefir, or yogurt.

13. Reduce Your Toxin Exposure:

• Pay attention to your surroundings and make an effort to limit your exposure to pollutants. This could entail selecting organic produce and utilizing natural cleaning supplies.

14. Life after Detoxification:

• After a detox, concentrate on leading a healthy, balanced lifestyle. Maintain your focus on eating good meals, getting regular exercise, and managing stress.

Recall that every person reacts differently to detoxification procedures, so it's important to pay attention to your body. Before making big dietary or lifestyle changes, it's best to speak with a healthcare provider if you have any underlying medical illnesses or concerns.

Conclusion

In summary, the body goes through a natural, continuous process called detoxification in which many organs and systems cooperate to get rid of pollutants. Even while the word "detox" is frequently linked to particular diets and cleanses, it's crucial to approach these practices cautiously and take into account each person's demands and health situation.

• Detox diets can take many different forms, from whole-food-based regimens to juice cleanses, and they are frequently advertised for their possible advantages, which include better digestion, more energy, and clearer skin. However, there is little scientific proof to support the effectiveness and safety of many detox diets, and there may be dangers associated with severe or protracted detoxification procedures.

• It's best to speak with a healthcare provider before starting a detox so they can offer you individualized advice depending on your goals and current state of health. Furthermore, emphasizing sustainable lifestyle habits can enhance general wellbeing and assist the body's natural detoxification processes. These practices include eating a balanced diet, drinking plenty of water, exercising frequently, reducing stress, and getting enough sleep.

Recall that the human body has developed sophisticated cleansing mechanisms. It is frequently more efficient and long-lasting to support these processes through good behaviors rather than depending on temporary, drastic methods. Make decisions that suit your unique requirements and preferences, with an emphasis on your long-term health and well-being.

THE END